BONE BROTH

Learn How Bone Broth Can Make Your Skin Glow, Improve your Health and Reverse Grey Hair - With Delicious Bone Broth Recipes!

BY
KATYA JOHANSSON

Copyright © 2016 by Katya Johansson.
All Rights Reserved.

TABLE OF CONTENTS

INTRODUCTION – MY STORY ... 1
CHAPTER 1: WHAT IS A BONE BROTH ? ... 2
   A Bone? Really? ... 2
CHAPTER 2: THE BONE BROTH DIET – THE SCIENCE BEHIND IT ... 5
   Broths, Bone Broth and Stocks ... 5
   What's the difference between stock, broth, and bone broth? ... 5
   why bone broths are good for you ... 6
CHAPTER 3: REASONS YOU SHOULD DRINK BONE BROTH EVERY DAY ... 8
   Bone broth patches up your gut ... 8
   Bone broth erases your wrinkles ... 10
   Bone broth aids you in losing weight fast ... 11
   Bone broth protects your joints ... 11
   Better Digestion ... 12
   Detox ... 13
   Marrow ... 14
   Minerals ... 15
   Other Benefits ... 16
CHAPTER 4: BONE BROTH RECIPES ... 18
   Making A Good Bone Broth ... 18
   Not sure what kind of bone to use? ... 18
   Cooking Recommendations ... 19
   Use Bone Broth With Your Next Fast ... 20
   Bone Broth Recipe: ... 21
CONCLUSION ... 23

Introduction – My Story

When I heard "bone broth" for the first time, I squeezed my face, and felt like Ew, "What? Why?"

I never knew what it meant, only that it sounded gross. However, I heard about it more and more from wellness websites, food bloggers and overall trendspotters

Here's what I can tell you: bone broth is a dressed-up stock. You can prepare it with animal bones — chicken, beef, turkey, whatsoever — just roast and simmer with veggies for hours. This is not a new food (grandma's have been preparing it for years).

The minerals and vitamins you derive from the broken-down bones have potent healing assets, and can assist in alleviating gut and joint pain, brighten skin, enhance your immune system, and give you a healthy hair.

Chapter 1: What Is A Bone Broth ?

Bone broth is a nutrient-dense meal. It's rich in magnesium and calcium, which is easily absorbed in the body. It's also enriched in glycine, amino acids and proline, which cannot be found in substantial amounts of meat which we largely consume. During the preparation period, if you want to speedily dissolve nutrients from the bone, all you have to do is to add vinegar. A small quantity of vinegar is required so as to not make it evident in taste.

Bone broths are really inexpensive and very easy to make. You can make Bone broths from the bones of fit animals like bison, beef, lamb, fish or poultry. Numerous food stores sell only the bones for at a cheap rate. At a native Chinese grocery within Toronto, you can get 3 chicken remains for as low as $1.50. Pork neck bones only cost $0.69/pound. This means that if you want to buy 3 pounds of bones, it would cost you about $2.10 for a big pot. You can use it in stews, soups, gravies and reductions. You can also use them to roast and braise meats, or for roasting or sautéing vegetables. If you drink a cup of hearty bone broth daily, it can help fight infection, enhance digestion, build muscle and reduce inflammation and joint pain all over the body.

A Bone? Really?

When you look at a bone, you will think that nothing good can come out of it. If you bite it, all you will achieve is getting your tooth sore, Lick it, and you will discover an unpleasant taste.

BONE BROTH

You begin to wonder the kind of nutrients that could perhaps be in there?

The answer is just about everything. Bones are a picture-perfect instance of why you shouldn't ever judge a book by the cover. Locked inside the hard shell is an abundance of vital nutrients – gut-healing proteins and anti-inflammatory, fats that are healthy, and a wealth of minerals waiting to be utilized. Even wild animals all over the world know this: they go for the bones each time they kill an animal.

An easy way to get to the nutrients within the bone is by preparing bone broth. The formulas are so easy that a child can do it. First, get some bones. Any kind of animal will do: the heads, feet, necks, backs, tails or knuckles, are all seamlessly good. Every now and then you can get parts like these from a farmer or butcher for free, or an extreme cut-price as "pet food." Remains from your last meal are good too. Prepare your broth with garnishes and seasonings though optional if you like them; also throw in whatsoever tastes good to you.

The result is going to be a clear, rich color which ranges from golden-yellow (chicken bones), translucent (fish bones) to deep brown (ruminant bones). If you add vegetables, this might affect the color; for instance, beets can turn it red. After staying some hours inside the fridge, the broth is going to solidify into the consistency of Jell-O: that is a sign that you have done it right. A layer of fat will appear at the top of the broth; if you are utilizing bones from hale and hearty animals, there is no reason for you not to enjoy this, but suppose you are trapped with grocery-store bones, wait until the stock has congealed to enable the tough fat scrape off easily.

Bone broth gives an amazing taste when utilized in stews or soups. The outstanding thing about it is the health benefits found in it.

Chapter 2: The Bone Broth Diet – The Science Behind It

Broths, Bone Broth and Stocks

Bone broths are of great importance among traditional foods providers. Preindustrial civilizations across the world have always placed specific emphasis on the preparation of a whole animal – and that comprises emphasis on u utilizing bones for preparing broth. In Asia, much emphasis is placed on broths and stocks prepared from fish bones and fish likewise beef bones for widespread soups like the Korean bone soup. Within Europe, broths and stocks have come to be the base of cooking and are been used not only for preparing stews and soups and stews, but also for making sauces, reductions and for braising meats and vegetables.

What's the difference between stock, broth, and bone broth?

Within traditional food circles you are going to hear a lot about broth, bone broth and stock – and how they are used interchangeably. Bone broth, stock and broth come from the same foundation: meat, water or bones (or even both), seasonings and vegetables. As you begin to cook it, the liquid typically skims and ultimately the solids are detached by straining the stock with a fine-mesh sieve orr usable coffee filter.

Broth is prepared with meat and contains little amount of bones (let your thoughts go over the bones in a whole fresh chicken). Broth is usually boiled over a little period of time (within 45 min to 2 hours). It's light in flavor, rich in protein and thin in texture.

Stock is typically prepared with bones contains a little amount of meat (let your thoughts go over the meat that stick to a beef neck bone). Most times the bones gets roasted prior to cooking them, and it's because it greatly enhances the flavor. Beef stocks, for instance, can produce a faint unpleasant flavor if the bones are not first roasted. Stock is naturally simmered for a modest amount of time (let's say 3 to 4 hours). Stock is one of the best source of gelatin.

Bone Broth is usually prepared with bones and contains a little amount of meat stuck to the bones. Just like stock, bones should be roasted first in order to enhance the taste of the bone broth. Bone broths are simmered for long periods of time (often 24 hours), with the sole aim of producing gelatin from collagen-rich joints and also to discharge minerals from the bones. When cooking has been completed, the bones are supposed to disintegrate when lightly pressed between your forefinger and thumb.

WHY BONE BROTHS ARE GOOD FOR YOU

Bone broths are extremely rich in protein, and can be a good source of minerals. Glycine assists the bodies cleansing process and is utilized in the synthesis of bile salts, hemoglobin and other natural body occurring chemicals. Glycine also aids digestion and the discharge of gastric acids. Proline,

BONE BROTH

particularly when combined with vitamin C, aids good skin health. Bone broths are rich in gelatin which might assist your skin health. Gelatin also aids digestive health, which enables it to play a crucial role within GAPS diet. And, lastly, if you have ever wondered why chicken soup is suitable for a cold, there is science behind it. Chicken broth prevents neutrophil migration; meaning that, it aids mitigate the effects of flu, colds, and upper respiratory infections. Pretty awesome, huh?

Chapter 3: Reasons You Should Drink Bone Broth Every Day

If you are combatting creep, weight, wrinkles, fatigue and many other signs of aging, I know that it is highly tempting to go for a false "fix"— an energy drink, a diet pill, or a shot of Botox. However, I have the right drug for you. It is one of the most potent healing and anti-aging food: bone broth.

Bone broth is in demand right now, with everybody from celebrities like Gwyneth Paltrow and Shailene Woodley and NBA stars frantic about it. But that is not the reason I ask my patients to consume this slow-simmered broth prepared from the bones of chicken, meat, fish or turkey.

As a matter of fact, I liked bone broth years prior to it becoming the "in thing." For over a decade ago, I found out the fat-melting and healing attributes of this liquid gold and made it the base of my weight loss and anti-aging transformation. In addition, I even drink it daily. Here's why.

Bone broth patches up your gut

Bone broth is filled with collagen, which transforms to gelatin when cooked — gelatin is among the most powerful gut healers around. Gelatin is laden with glycine, a potent anti-inflammatory amino acid, and it is rich in other therapeutic nutrients which includes proline, magnesium and arginine.

BONE BROTH

Gelatin's gut-healing attributes are very vital. In order to be healthy and slim, your gut needs to be rock-solid. As a matter of fact, from my experience as a clinician who concentrates on transforming overweight and sick patients into slender healthy individuals, I can only tell you that there is nothing more significant to your health than having a strong gut. Here is the story.

Your gut is host to trillions of microbes that experts call the microbiome. Look at this microbiome as an ecological unit — one that is either out of balance or in balance. If it is in balance, you've got a wide variety of good microbes and some few bad ones. If it is out of balance, there are two dangerous things involved:

The bad microbes can increase speedily, tossing out poisonous chemicals.

Small intestinal bacterial overgrowth (SIBO) can happen. Within SIBO, microbes overpopulate your gut, thus overpowering it.

There're numerous reasons your gut can be out of balance. Here're some of the key ones:

The use of Antibiotics, which exterminates trillions of good microbes.

Eating the wrong foods, which gets them starved.

Stress, this poisons their environment.

NSAIDS, Antacids, and other gut-altering treatments, which can change the "chemistry" of their ecological unit in destructive ways.

When bad microbes advance too much within your gut, or when good microbes increase rapidly, they yield chemicals that can cause swelling. This swelling in turn damages your intestinal wall, bringing about a "leaky gut or intestinal permeability." This allows toxins, bacteria and waste to drip into your bloodstream and being identified by your immune system as alien to your body system, thus triggering a flood of inflammatory chemicals, even though there is no more war to fight. This in turn will cause chronic swelling — and it is a known fact that this chronic swelling lies beneath every ailment of aging, from diabetes and obesity to cancer and heart disease.

Gelatin aids in transforming a leaky gut to a strong barricade, heal chronic swelling and make your whole body healthier. As a result, you will shed extra pounds easily, feel very energetic, and even notice that skin difficulties like eczema will begin to clear up.

BONE BROTH ERASES YOUR WRINKLES

High-end wrinkle ointments are filled with collagen, which strengthens and firms the cells within your skin. Though, it is far more effective to build collagen from within. Whenever you consume bone broth, it's like mainlining the modules of collagen to your skin.

Bone broth contains hyaluronic acid, which will hydrate your skin and erase wrinkles. (Babies' skin are filled with hyaluronic acid, which is the reason it is very soft.) Again, you can either pay huge sums of money for skin ointments containing this wrinkle blaster — or just feed it directly to your cells, the natural way.

BONE BROTH

BONE BROTH AIDS YOU IN LOSING WEIGHT FAST

Unlike the moist broth you get in cans, bone broth is hearty, rich and satisfying. If you drink a cup of bone broth, you will feel like you have consumed a full meal, even though you are merely taking around 50 to 60 calories. The bottom line is that, you will not get cravings, even if you drastically reduce your food intake.

If my patients want to lose weight quickly, I ask them to do 2 semi-fasting in a week, eating nothing but bone broth on those days. Some of them originally are not sure they can do it. But, they quickly find out that the weight dissolves right off them, and now they are astonished at how efficiently bone broth halts their yearnings for junk food and sugar.

BONE BROTH PROTECTS YOUR JOINTS

Your joints comprise cartilage, a slick Teflon-like layer that permits the joints to slide over one another without crunching. Likewise, you can find cartilage in animal bones. Cartilage is rich in collagen and is also filled with chondroitin sulfate and glucosamine— the same nutrients that many physicians prescribe as supplements in keeping the joints healthy and young.

A random clinical trial in the year 2015 established that oral glucosamine and chondroitin were as effective as the arthritis medication Celebrex in decreasing swelling, pain and functional restrictions instigated by knee osteoarthritis. And because they are natural nutrients, chondroitin and glucosamine have a flawless safety profile — unlike the potentially dangerous drug Celebrex.

You can prepare bone broth within your own kitchen

Here is one of the paramount things about bone broth: You do not require prescriptions for it! All you require is a slow cooker and a big pot, numerous pounds of bones, some vegetables and spices, and some hours to allow your broth cook.

Think about it: What other medication can assist you in losing weight, look younger, provide you with more energy, patch up your joints, and wipe out your wrinkles, all without a prescription, a trip to the medicine store or side effects other than a happy, warm, fulfilled feeling? This is why bone broth happens to be the base of my anti-aging and weight-loss transformation… and why you should emulate me and utilize it as the base of your health regimen as well.

Dr Petrucci, M.S., N.D., who happens to be the author of Kellyann's Bone Broth Diet. A natural weight loss and anti-aging makeover expert, Dr. Petrucci has a private practice in Birmingham, Michigan area and is a celebrity doctor in New Los Angeles and York City. She is also a board-certified naturopathic doctor and a certified nutrition specialist.

BETTER DIGESTION

Nature seldom make foods that're hale and hearty for one reason only, and bone broth is not excluded. It helps keep your knees free from worrying crunchy noises each time you move, it also aids digestion in a number of ways.

Glycine, for instance, is useful because it fuels the production of stomach acid. If you judge from the millions of dollars Americans devote on antacids yearly, you might begin to think that this's the last thing we require, as a matter of fact, acid reflux might be an issue of too little or less stomach acid. A stomach acid shortage leaves your food half-digested in your stomach, and the stress from your stomach [being so full] can therefore force acid into the esophagus.

By making your body secrete additional stomach acid, glycine can assist in preventing or treating this painful and dangerous problem. Thus making bone broth a delightful supplemental meal for anyone suffering from IBS or acid.

Glycine is also a vital component of bile acid, which is needed for fat digestion within the small intestine, and also it helps to maintain a healthy blood cholesterol level. Especially for those who're new to Paleo and are switching from a carb-based meal to a fat-based meal, this has the all it takes to keep the digestive procedure running more smoothly.

Glycine is not the only valuable protein for gut health. Glutamine, another amino acid established in bone broth, is a typical remedy for "leaky gut," that dangerous and unpleasant condition where the barricade between the rest of your body and your gut is not working well, thus letting molecules that are supposed to stay within the gut to cross over to the bloodstream and possibly set off a flow of autoimmune responses. Glutamine aids in maintaining the functions of the intestinal wall, stopping this destruction from happening.

Detox

Glycine helps in cleansing —because your body system has its own detoxification system: The liver. Glycine provides the liver a hand up in getting rid of anything dangerous from the body –

for instance, in one rat study, rats that were fed glycine showed noteworthy advances in recovering from alcohol-induced fatty liver illness compared to rats that were not.

Glycine is also very necessary for the production of uric acid and glutathione, the body's most important endogenous antioxidants. As labeled in the article on antioxidants, the boosting production of internally produced antioxidants is more useful in decreasing oxidative stress than consuming Vitamin C or various antioxidant supplements.

Another detox-related advantage is that glycine assists in clearing out surplus methionine, another amino acid seen in muscle meat and eggs. Methionine is a necessary amino acid, but when you have it in abundance, it can raise the blood levels of homocysteine, however the process of breaking down homocysteine rises the body's need for vitamin B. Glycine from cartilage and broths can help in breaking down homocysteine without needing B vitamins. This is an impeccable instance of the wisdom of traditional beliefs in consuming all parts of an animal: the proteins found within the muscle meat and the proteins within the connective tissue balance one other for optimum nutrition.

Marrow

All kind of broth is healthy, but broth prepared with marrow bones are particularly valuable because you the marrow contains so much good stuffs just like the bones have good stuffs in them. Whenever you find animals tearing through the bones of another dead animal, it is the marrow they are after.

BONE BROTH

Vultures even fly up with bones only to smash on rocks, and then plunge down to taste delicious interior.

The bone marrow is very delicious. It is usually touted as enormously nutritious– and it possibly is, given that it is an organ meat and organ meats tend to have exceptional nutritional value. The Bone marrow is a vital part of the immune system, and it contains all types of cells that are essential for bone growth and immune function. Regrettably, there's no definite nutritional exploration of it yet, that's why few people are eating it. It's a fact that it is filled with monounsaturated fat, and Dr. Weston A. Price talked about numerous traditional cultures who see it as a consecrated food for fertility nourishment; unfortunately, we have to wait till a more thorough nutritional exploration is available.

MINERALS

Apart from the benefits of all the sugars and proteins, and the nutrients that may be hiding within the marrow, bone broth is very high in minerals. Land animals and Bones are rich in magnesium, calcium, potassium and phosphorus, also fish bones contain iodine. We are aware that some of this mineral content leaks out into the water, because the bones are demineralized and crumbly when the broth is cooked – often they are very weak that they are going to fall apart if you apply pressure on them. If you utilize smaller bones, like fish or chicken, they will occasionally dissolve into the stock.

Unfortunately, it is not possible to get an exact estimation of how much of these minerals within the broth because every batch of bone is different. The nutritional content of the broth will be influenced heavily on how the animal was preserved, how many bones were utilized, what its diet was like, whether there was any meat left on them, what portion of the animal the bones came from, how long were they cooked, and at what level of temperature. In short, it is not possible to give you a list of "bone broth nutrition info."

There are some ways to make the most of the mineral content. The coolest is to add some tablespoons of something acidic to the broth prior to you turning on the heat. If you have once put an egg into a glass of vinegar, then you've seen this work: the shell comprise of calcium carbonate, so it fades away and melts, and the egg is held by nothing but the membrane.

Another meek way to get the most nourishment from your broth is to consume only the bones. After cooking it for a long time, small bones are not hard at all; they have this texture that's just a little tougher than crunchy nut butter. If you cannot handle them straight, the alternative will be to grind them in a blender and take them as supplements.

OTHER BENEFITS

Just like the major merits above, there is also a grab-bag of various other explanations to get your broth in. In general, all proteins within bone broth are intensely anti-inflammatory. This might actually be why some are so useful in treating osteoarthritis (this is an inflammatory autoimmune illness), leaky gut (an inflammatory predecessor to autoimmune illnesses), and other prolonged inflammatory circumstances like fatty liver or joint pain disease.

BONE BROTH

Another anti-inflammatory value of the proteins within bone broth is rapid recovery from wound. Under stress of a disease or injury, the body requires more amino acids – that's why a lot of them are regarded as "provisionally important" even though technically they are not obligated in the diet because it is likely to make them from additional sources. During periods of stress or increased physical demand, the body requires a lot of amino acids than produces, so they do turn out to be "vital," and getting a lot it can hasten recovery.

The most notable instances of this are glutamine and arginine, both discovered in bone broth. Supplementary dietary arginine assists in speeding wound healing by being supportive to the formation of collagen. Glutamine also assists in reducing healing time within hospital patients, and the recovery period within athletes on an extreme training routine.

One more fringe benefit of broth is glycine and it's is an inhibitory neurotransmitter, which means that it assists you in relaxing. One trial discovered that glycine supplements improves the quality of sleep and reduces daytime sleepiness. So a mug of bone broth may just be the ticket you need in winding down after a long day.

Just so you know, the amino acids within gelatin improves the appearance of your hair and skin. Gelatin-rich broths help to build connective tissues, which makes the skin to be healthier and smoother (fewer wrinkles, less cellulite). There is also some indication that it reduces the signs of aging, but be cautious when digging for the evidence: most of the investigation into this is being funded by industry promoters, so it isn't very reliable.

Chapter 4: Bone Broth Recipes

Making A Good Bone Broth

When gathering bones, go for assortment.

The reason is because the marrow discovered within the bones is either red marrow or yellow marrow. Yellow marrow is discovered in the central portion of long bones. This is where fats are deposited.

Red marrow is discovered in flat bones. Which includes:

Sternum

Hip bone

Ribs

Skull

Vertebrae

Scapula

The ends of the long bones

Red marrow is so appreciated because blood stem cells are discovered there. Whenever you consume a broth prepared with a decent source of red marrow, you are taking in all those stem cell elements that eventually build the strength in your body and support your own immune function.

Not Sure What Kind Of Bone To Use?

BONE BROTH

You can use any type. You can even utilize a variety of different animals. Just ensure that all the bones are obtained from animals that're grass-fed and organic or free-range and pastured. Bear in mind that everything the animal ate, where it lived and how it lived, all influence health benefits of your broth.

You can buy bones ready to cook, or you can gather bones from meals and stock them in your freezer until you have amassed enough to build a good stock. Bear in mind to only utilize feet and bones from animals that are free-range or grass-fed.

Ensure that the bones particularly large bones, are cut into little pieces. This decreases the cooking time and it enables more material to turn into a part of the broth.

COOKING RECOMMENDATIONS

1. Place the bones into a big stock pot and cover it with water.

2. Add 2 tablespoon of wine or apple cider vinegar to water before cooking. This will assist in pulling out significant nutrients within the bones.

3. Fill the stock pot with clean water. Allow the water to boil.

4. Heat it slowly. Bring it to a boiling point and then reduce the heat to simmer for at least 6 hours. Take away filth as it arises.

5. Cook slow and long. Chicken bones can cook for about 6-48 hours while Beef bones can cook for up to 12-72 hours. A slow and long cook time is essential to completely extract the nutrients around and within the bone.

After cooking, the broth is going to cool off and a layer of fat will solidify on top. This coating shields the broth underneath. Get rid of this layer only when you're ready to consume the broth.

Eat the broth within 3 days or freeze it for later use. Sip on the broth or utilize it as the core in a nutrient-dense stew.

USE BONE BROTH WITH YOUR NEXT FAST

During fasting, the body gets little nourishment from meals. Because of this, muscle tissues can break down.

Whenever glycine is eaten, it prevents or limits the breakdown of protein tissue, such as muscle.

Glycine is utilized for gluconeogenesis, where the liver creates sugar fuel for the body to burn if there is no presence of glucose.

Glycine is also essential to cleanse the body of chemicals. This is because glycine is a predecessor amino acid for glutathione, which is a key detoxifying and antioxidant agent within the body.

Glycine is regarded as an inhibitory neurotransmitter. It improves sleep, as well as enhances performance and memory.

BONE BROTH

BONE BROTH RECIPE:

Ingreddients:

3-4 pounds beef marrow and knuckle bones

2 pounds meaty bones such as short ribs

½ cup raw apple cider vinegar

4 quarts filtered water

3 celery stalks, halved

3 carrots, halved

3 onions, quartered

Handful of fresh parsley

Sea salt

Method Of Preparation:

Place bones in a pot or a crockpot, add apple cider vinegar and water, and let the mixture sit for 1 hour so the vinegar can leach the mineral out of the bones.

Add more water if needed to cover the bones.

Add the vegetables bring to a boil and skim the scum from the top and discard.

Reduce to a low simmer, cover, and cook for 24-72 hours (if you're not comfortable leaving the pot to simmer overnight, turn off the heat and let it sit overnight, then turn it back on and let simmer all day the next day)

During the last 10 minutes of cooking, throw in a handful of fresh parsley for added flavor and minerals.

Let the broth cool and strain it, making sure all marrow is knocked out of the marrow bones and into the broth.

Add sea salt to taste and drink the broth as is or store in fridge up to 5 to 7 days or freezer up to 6 months for use in soups or stews.

Conclusion

The old song – "Dem bones, dem bones, dry bones" – got it wrong. Bones are not dry; when prepared properly, they are one of the best nutrient-dense foodstuffs you can consume. And the price is pocket friendly, too: think of the many bones we throw out weekly.

Utilizing those bones will save you a substantial amount of money, because it stretches a roasting chicken or a leg of lamb into not one, but two high value sources of fat and protein. Drink up!

www.ingramcontent.com/pod-product-compliance
Lightning Source LLC
Chambersburg PA
CBHW070309190526
45169CB00004B/1562